Contents

INTRODUCTION

Cutting again on carbs isn't always very complex.

Just update the sugars and starches on your
weight loss program with veggies, meat, fish,
eggs, nuts and fat.

Seems pretty straightforward, unless you don't
devour meat.

Conventional low-carb diets rely heavily on meat,
which makes them flawed for vegetarians.

However, this does not want to be the case.

Everyone can follow a low-carb eating regimen,
even vegetarians and vegans.

This book suggests you the way to do it and delicious recipes to do with.

WHY LOW-CARB?

In the beyond 12 years, at the least 23 studies have proven that low-carb diets allow you to lose weight (without calorie counting).

One of the primary motives is that those diets can substantially lessen urge for food, making you consume fewer energy without having to consciously try and devour much less.

Low-carb diets additionally enhance health in other ways.

They are very powerful at reducing dangerous stomach fats, and generally tend to reduce triglycerides and raise HDL (the "appropriate") cholesterol significantly. They also generally tend to lower blood stress and blood sugar ranges.

Although low-carb diets are not important for anyone, they are able to have important fitness blessings for human beings humans with weight problems, metabolic syndrome, kind 2 diabetes and certain neurological disorders.

A low-carb vegan food regimen can be very healthful as nicely. Studies on eco-atkins (vegan, 26% of calories as carbs) have shown that this sort of weight loss plan is tons healthier than a everyday low-fat weight-reduction plan, in addition to a low-fats vegetarian weight loss

plan.

DIFFERENT TYPES OF VEGETARIANS

There are several one-of-a-kind forms of

vegetarians. None of them devour meat or fish.

The most not unusual sorts are lacto-ovo

vegetarians and vegans.

Lacto-ovo vegetarians (or honestly "vegetarians")

consume dairy merchandise and eggs, but vegans

do no longer eat any animal-derived foods.

DAIRY PRODUCTS AND EGGS ARE LOW IN CARBS

Eggs and dairy merchandise, without brought sugar, are low in carbs, but excessive in both protein and fats. For vegetarians (now not vegans), they're best for an extremely low-carb diet.

Eggs: Contain best hint quantities of carbs. Choose pastured, omega-three-enriched or free-range eggs if you can.

Yogurt, Greek yogurt and kefir: Choose unsweetened, full-fat variations. Find ones with live cultures for an additional probiotic benefit.

Grass-fed butter: Butter from grass-fed cows is healthy, and best carefully on a low-carb weight loss program.

Cheese: Highly nutrient-dense and attractive, and can be utilized in all varieties of recipes.

These meals are also wealthy in diet B12, which isn't located in plant meals. Vegetarians can get all the B12 they want from these ingredients, while vegans want to complement.

LOW-CARB FRIENDLY PLANT FOODS (FOR BOTH VEGETARIANS AND VEGANS)

There is virtually a big style of low-carb ingredients from plants.

Many of these ingredients also are excessive in protein and fat.

Vegetables: Many vegetables are low in carbs. This consists of tomatoes, onions, cauliflower, eggplant, bell peppers, broccoli and Brussels sprouts.

Fruits: Berries like strawberries and blueberries may be eaten on a low-carb weight-reduction plan. Depending on how many carbs you want to consume, other fruits can be acceptable as well.

Fatty culmination: Avocados and olives are fairly wholesome. They are low in carbs however high in fat.

Nuts and seeds: Nuts and seeds are low in carbs, however excessive in protein and fat. This includes almonds, walnuts, macadamia nuts, peanuts and pumpkin seeds.

Soy: Foods like tofu and tempeh are excessive in protein and fats, but low in carbs. This makes them ideal on a low-carb vegetarian/vegan weight loss program.

Legumes: Some legumes, including inexperienced beans, chick peas and others.

Healthy fats: Extra virgin olive oil, avocado oil and coconut oil.

Chia seeds: Most of the carbs in chia seeds are fiber, so almost all of the usable calories in them come from protein and fat.

Dark chocolate: If you choose darkish chocolate with a excessive (70-85%+) cocoa content material, then it is going to be low in carbs however excessive in fats.

HOW MANY CARBS SHOULD YOU EAT?

There isn't any fixed definition of exactly what "low carb" manner.

It is crucial to experiment and discern out a way to suit your carb intake to your personal dreams and choices.

That being said, those pointers are reasonable:

100-a hundred and fifty grams in keeping with day: This is a respectable renovation variety, and is right for those who exercise plenty.

50-100 grams per day: This should cause automatic weight loss, and is a superb preservation variety for folks who do not exercise that tons.

20-50 grams in keeping with day: With a carb intake this low, you have to shed pounds quickly without experiencing much starvation. This carb variety have to placed you into ketosis.

Vegetarians may want to without problems move into the lowest variety, however this sort of weight loss plan would be impractical for vegans.

The 100-150 gram range would be extra suitable

for vegans.

It is recommended to apply a nutrition tracker

(like Cron-o-meter) for at the least a few

days/weeks at the same time as you're nice-

tuning your carbohydrate consumption and

ensuring to get sufficient protein and fat.

A SAMPLE MENU FOR A LOW-CARB VEGETARIAN DIET

This is a one-week pattern menu for a vegetarian

(now not vegan) weight-reduction plan this is low

in carbs.

You can adapt this primarily based in your very own desires and preferences.

Monday

Breakfast: Eggs and greens, fried in olive oil.

Lunch: Four bean salad with olive oil, and a handful of nuts.

Dinner: Cheesy cauliflower bake (gratin) with broccoli and tofu.

Tuesday

Breakfast: Full-fats yoghurt and berries.

Lunch: Leftover cauliflower bake from the night time before.

Dinner: Grilled portabello mushrooms, with buttered vegetables and avocado.

Wednesday

Breakfast: Smoothie with coconut milk and blueberries.

Lunch: Carrot and cucumber sticks with hummus dip, and a handful of nuts.

Dinner: Tempeh stir fry, with cashew nuts and greens.

Thursday

Breakfast: Omelet with vegetables, fried in olive oil.

Lunch: Leftover stir fry from dinner the night time before.

Dinner: Chilli beans with sour cream, cheese and salsa.

Friday

Breakfast: Full-fats yoghurt and berries.

Lunch: Leafy greens and hard-boiled eggs with some olive oil and a handful of nuts.

Dinner: Feta cheese salad with pumpkin seeds and macadamia nuts, drizzled with olive oil.

Saturday

Breakfast: Fried eggs with baked beans and avocado.

Lunch: Carrot and cucumber sticks with hummus dip, and a handful of nuts.

Dinner: Eggplant moussaka.

Sunday

Breakfast: Strawberry smoothie with full-fat yogurt and nuts.

Lunch: Leftover moussaka from the night time before.

Dinner: Asparagus, spinach and feta quiche (with or without egg).

LOW CARB VEGETARIAN DIET COOKBOOK

Easy Keto Creamed Spinach

This makes a total of three servings of Easy Keto Creamed Spinach.Each serving comes out to be one hundred sixty five Calories, 13.22g Fats, 3.63g Net Carbs, and seven.33g Protein.

Ingredients

• 10 oz. Frozen spinach

• three tablespoons Parmesan cheese

• 3 oz. Cream cheese

- 2 tablespoons butter cream

- ¼ teaspoon garlic powder

- ¼ teaspoon onion powder

- Salt and pepper to flavor

Instructions

1. Defrost frozen spinach within the microwave. Add to pan on medium-excessive warmth and permit extra water boil off.

2. Add seasoning and cream cheese to the pan. Stir collectively until cream cheese has melted.

3. Add sour cream and parmesan and mix together nicely till the creamed spinach is thickened.

EGGPLANT AND WILLIAM MAXWELL AITKEN ALFREDO

This makes a complete of 6 servings of Eggplant and Sir Francis Bacon Alfredo. Each serving comes out to be 564 Calories, fifty one.25g Fats, 6.34g Net Carbs, and 16.7g Protein.

Ingredients

- 1 pound bacon

- 1½ pounds eggplant

- 1 cup heavy whipping cream

- 2 tablespoons butter

- 2 cloves garlic, grated

- 1 tablespoon white wine

- 1 tablespoon lemon juice

- 1 cup shredded Parmesan cheese

Instructions

1. Chop up the bacon and fry over medium heat in a huge skillet.

2. When the bacon has rendered out and becomes crisp then dispose of it from the pan and drain on paper towels. Save all of the bacon grease.

3. Peel and julienne the eggplant. Cook it within the bacon grease till it softens. In the photographs you may see that I changed pans

due to the fact the primary one wasn't going to be huge sufficient. You can use the identical pan if it is big enough for all the eggplant.

4. As the eggplant chefs it's going to absorb all of the bacon grease. Create a properly within the center then upload the 2 tablespoons of butter. Stir all the noodles so that they turn out to be lined with the melted butter then blend within the grated garlic.

5. Pour the cup of heavy whipping cream into the pan. Add the white wine and lemon juice then stir collectively.

6. Add the cup of shredded Parmesan cheese and stir.

7. Mix in about half of the bacon.

8. Serve with the ultimate bacon sprinkled on top. Chopped up clean basil additionally makes a wonderful garnish.

KETO MUG LASAGNA

This makes a complete of 1servings of Keto Mug Lasagna. Each serving comes out to be 318 Calories, 23.54g Fats, five.39g Net Carbs, and 20.45g Protein.

Ingredients

- 1/3 (65 g) zucchini

- three tablespoons Rao's marinara

- 2 tablespoons entire milk ricotta

- three oz. Entire milk mozzarella

Instructions

1. Slice the zucchini into paper thin rounds. You can use a virtually sharp knife, or a mandolin.

2. In the bottom of your dish upload a tablespoon of the marinara.

3. Layer on some of the zucchini.

4. Carefully unfold out 1 tablespoon of ricotta.

5. Add some other tablespoon of marinara.

6. Layer on the second one layer of zucchini, another tablespoon of ricotta, any leftover

zucchini, and then the ultimate tablespoon of marinara.

7. Top with the mozzarella.

8. Microwave for 3-4 minutes, depending at the strength of your microwave. You can sprinkle on a touch oregano or Parmesan cheese if you want.

FLUFFY BUTTERMILK PANCAKES

This makes a complete of one servings of Fluffy Buttermilk Pancakes. Each serving comes out to be 422 Calories, 19.28g Fats, 13.01g Net Carbs, and 32.75g Protein.

Ingredients

- 2 huge eggs, separated

- ½ cup liquid egg whites or egg replacement*

- ½ cup buttermilk

- 1 teaspoon vanilla extract

- 1 tablespoon protein powder

- ¼ cup coconut flour

- 1 teaspoon baking powder

- Dash of cinnamon

- 1 packet of Stevia

- Butter or oil for cooking

Instructions

1. Beat your two separated egg whites with a pinch of salt till smooth peaks have formed

2. Mix all different ingredients in another bowl.

3. In any other bowl, whisk dry ingredients.

4. Add dry components to wet and mix until properly combined.

5. Fold whipped egg whites into your batter, making sure now not to deflate the whites

6. Preheat a non-stick skillet over medium-low warmth

7. Lightly grease your pan with butter or cooking spray

8. Pour ¼ cup of batter into your pan, moving barely to distribute evenly.

9. Cook until bubbles are seen on the pinnacle, flip, and cook the alternative facet till golden brown.

ASPARAGUS FRIES WITH RED PEPPER AIOLI

This makes a complete of two massive servings of Parmesan Asparagus Fries with Roasted Red Pepper Aioli. Each serving comes out to be 453.65 Calories, 33.63 g Fat, 5.51 g Net Carbs, and 19.14 g Protein.

Ingredients

- 10 medium asparagus spears

- ½ cup shredded Parmesan cheese

- 2 tablespoons chopped parsley

- ½ teaspoon garlic powder

- ¼ cup almond flour

- ½ teaspoon smoked paprika

- 2 large eggs

- three tablespoon mayonnaise

- 1 tablespoon finely chopped roasted red pepper

Instructions

1. Heat oven to 425°F and wash the asparagus spears. In a food processor, combine the shredded Parmesan cheese, parsley, garlic powder, and pulse until pleasant.

2. Add almond flour to the meals processor and pulse a couple of times to combine. Transfer to a medium sized shallow dish. Stir in smoked paprika.

3. In a medium bowl, beat two eggs until they come to be frothy. The eggs will adhere to the asparagus a good deal better if they may be beaten nicely. Transfer egg to a medium length shallow dish.

4. Dip asparagus spears inside the egg mixture first. Holding the spear above the Parmesan flour aggregate, lightly sprinkle whilst turning until the asparagus is gently covered. Make certain to maintain the asparagus from touching the flour mix or the egg will reason it to grow to be too wet and clumpy. Repeat with each spear.

5. Place coated asparagus tightly spaced on a baking sheet and pinnacle with the leftover parmesan flour mixture. Bake until the coating begins to brown and the asparagus is only barely soft, about 10 mins.

6. In a small bowl blend the finely chopped roasted pink pepper and mayonnaise.

7. Chill the sauce inside the fridge and permit the flavors to combine. Stir nicely before serving.

8. Once asparagus fries are crisp and brown, eliminate from the oven and serve warm with the dip!

5 MINUTE KETO PIZZA

This makes a total of one 5 Minute Keto Pizza. Each pizza comes out to be 459 Calories, 35g Fats, 3.5g Carbs, and 27g Protein.

Ingredients

• Pizza Crust

• 2 large Eggs

- 2 tbsp. Parmesan Cheese

- 1 tbsp. Psyllium Husk Powder

- 1/2 tsp. Italian Seasoning

- Salt to Taste

- 2 tsp. Frying Oil (I use bacon fats)

- Toppings

- 1.5 ounces. Mozzarella Cheese

- three tbsp. Rao's Tomato Sauce

- 1 tbsp. Freshly Chopped Basil

Instructions

1. In a bowl or container, use an immersion blender to combine collectively all pizza crust ingredients.

2. Heat frying oil in a pan till hot, then spoon the combination into the pan. Spread out right into a circle.

3. Once edges are browned, flip and cook dinner for 30-60 seconds on the opposite facet. Turn the range off, and flip the broiler on.

4. Add tomato sauce and cheese, then broil for 1-2 minutes or till cheese is bubbling.

CHARRED VEGGIE AND FRIED GOAT CHEESE SALAD

This makes 2 servings of Charred Veggie and Fried Goat Cheese Salad. Each serving comes out to be 350 Calories, 27.61 g Fat, 7.08 g Net Carbs, and 16.09 g Protein.

Ingredients

• 2 tablespoons poppy seeds

• 2 tablespoons sesame seeds

• 1 teaspoon onion flakes

• 1 teaspoon garlic flakes

• four ounces goat cheese, reduce into 4 ½ in thick medallions

- 1 medium red bell pepper, seeds removed, reduce into 8 portions

- ½ cup sliced infant portobello mushrooms

- four cups arugula, divided between two bowls

- 1 tablespoon avocado oil

Instructions

1. Combine the poppy and sesame seeds, onion, and garlic flakes in a small dish.

2. Coat every piece of goat cheese on both aspects. Plate and location in the fridge until you're prepared to fry the cheese.

3. Prepare a skillet with nonstick spray and warmth to medium. Char the peppers and

mushrooms on each aspects, simply until the portions begin to darken and the pepper softens. Add to the bowls of arugula.

4. Place the bloodless goat cheese inside the skillet and fry on each side for approximately 30 seconds. This melts quick so be mild as you turn each piece!

5. Add the cheese to the salad and drizzle with avocado oil. Serve warm!

KETO ZUCCHINI BREAD WITH WALNUTS

This makes a total of sixteen servings of Keto Zucchini Bread with Walnut Crust. Each slice comes out to be 200.13 Calories, 18.83g Fats, 2.6g Net Carbs, and 5.59g Protein.

Ingredients

- three massive eggs

- ½ cup olive oil

- 1 teaspoon vanilla extract

- 2 half cups almond flour

- 1 half cups erythritol

- ½ teaspoon salt

- 1 half of teaspoons baking powder

- ½ teaspoon nutmeg

- 1 teaspoon ground cinnamon

- ¼ teaspoon floor ginger

- 1 cup grated zucchini

- ½ cup chopped walnuts

Instructions

1. Preheat oven to 350°F. Whisk together the eggs, oil, and vanilla extract.Set to the facet.

2. In any other bowl, mix together the almond flour, erythritol, salt, baking powder, nutmeg, cinnamon, and ginger. Set to the facet.

3. Using a cheesecloth or paper towel, take the zucchini and squeeze out the excess water.

4. Then, whisk the zucchini into the bowl with the eggs.

5. Slowly add the dry substances into the egg aggregate using a hand mixer until fully blended.

6. Lightly spray a 9x5 loaf pan, and spoon inside the zucchini bread mixture.

7. Then, spoon in the chopped walnuts on top of the zucchini bread. Press walnuts into the batter the use of a spatula.

8. Bake for 60-70 mins at 350°F or till the walnuts on pinnacle look browned.

PUMPKIN SPICED FRENCH TOAST

This makes a total of two servings. Each serving comes out to be 429.73 Calories, 36.7g Fats, 7.33g Net Carbs, and 13.36g Protein.

Ingredients

- 4 slices pumpkin bread

- 1 large egg

- 2 tablespoons cream

- ½ teaspoon vanilla extract

- 1/eight teaspoon orange extract

- ¼ teaspoon pumpkin pie spice

- 2 tablespoons butter

Instructions

1. Let the bread dry out overnight in open air after you've got sliced it.

2. Mix together egg, extracts, and pumpkin pie spice. Let the bread soak on both sides in the aggregate.

3. Heat butter in pan till nearly browned, then upload bread slices. Flip when browned and preserve to cook till browned on both sides.

4. Serve with keto maple syrup and some extra powdered swerve.

CHEESY CAULIFLOWER CASSEROLE

This makes a total of 8 servings of Cheesy Cauliflower Casserole Each serving comes out to be 135.13 Calories, 10.48g Fats, 4.47g Net Carbs, and 5.42g Protein.

Ingredients

- 1 medium head of cauliflower

- ½ medium onion, chopped

- 1 cup sour cream

- 1 cup shredded cheddar cheese

- Salt and pepper to flavor

- The Execution

Instructions

1. Chop up your cauliflower into chew-length pieces, region it right into a casserole dish.

2. Dice up your onions and add it to the cauliflower.

3. Pour in your sour cream and cheese into the dish.

4. Mix it all together!

5. Bake at 350°F for 30 minutes.

ZUCCHINI RIBBONS WITH AVOCADO WALNUT PESTO

This makes a total of two servings of Zucchini Ribbons with Avocado Walnut Pesto. Each serving comes out to be 325.5 Calories, 26.08 g Fat, 11.46g Net Carbs, and 10.65g Protein.

Ingredients

• Zucchini Ribbons

- 3 medium zucchini

- ½ teaspoon salt

- Avocado Walnut Pesto

- ½ big avocado

- 1 cup sparkling basil leaves

- ¼ cup walnuts

- 2 cloves garlic, peeled

- ½ massive lemon

- ¼ cup grated Parmesan cheese

- ½ cup water, if needed*

Other

- 1 tablespoon olive oil

- five-6 sparkling basil leaves to garnish

- Salt and pepper to flavor

Optional: Italian seasoning*

Instructions

1. Cut the zucchini into delicate ribbons with a vegetable peeler or mandolin slicer, being cautious to prevent peeling once you attain the seeds.

2. Place the ribbons in a colander and toss with salt. Let stand even as you prepare the avocado pesto

3. Gather the avocado walnut pesto components. This consists of avocado, basil, walnuts, garlic, lemon, and cheese.

4. Add all elements into the meals processor and blend until the sauce is easy. Add water to skinny the sauce as needed.

5. Grease a skillet with 1 tablespoon olive oil and bring to medium heat.

6. Sauté zucchini ribbons for 3-5 mins or till they're simply beginning to melt. Remove from warmth.

7. Spoon pesto onto zucchini ribbons and gently toss to coat.

8. Plate in two portions of extraordinarily swirled vegetable ribbons. Garnish with fresh basil and grated Parmesan cheese.

GARLIC AND HERB MONKEY "BREAD"

This makes a total of three servings of Garlic Herb Monkey "Bread". Each serving comes out to be 194 Calories, 14.23 g Fat, 5.73 g Net Carbs, and 8 g Protein.

Ingredients

- 2 baby eggplants, ends eliminated and cubed

- ¾ cup shredded mozzarella cheese

- 1 teaspoon garlic powder

- ¼ teaspoon dried basil

- 2 tablespoons butter, melted

- 1 tablespoon chopped clean basil

- 3 mini Bundt pans

Instructions

1. Heat oven to 375°F. Combine the garlic powder and dried basil and add to melted butter.

2. Layer 7-10 cubes of eggplant inside the backside of each mini Bundt pan.

3. Sprinkle a layer of mozzarella cheese over every layer of eggplant and drizzle with about 1 teaspoon of the butter garlic combination. Don't

worry approximately being specific as it will all bake collectively!

4. Follow with another layer of eggplant, then cheese, and any closing garlic butter.

5. Top with the closing cheese and bake for about 20 minutes or until cheese is brown.

6. Let cool for 5 minutes before casting off from the pans. Serve warm with low-carb marinara sauce!

CINNAMON ROLL "OATMEAL"

This makes 6 total servings of Cinnamon Roll "Oatmeal". Each serving comes out to be 368.83

Calories, 34.43g Fats, 4.08g Net Carbs, and 5.85g

Protein.

Ingredients

- 1 cup beaten pecans

- 1/3 cup flax seed meal

- 1/three cup chia seeds

- ½ cup rice cauliflower (~ 3 oz.)

- 3 ½ cups coconut milk

- ¼ cup heavy cream

- 3 oz. Cream cheese

- 3 tablespoons butter

- 1 ½ teaspoons cinnamon

- 1 teaspoon maple flavor

- ½ teaspoon vanilla

- ¼ teaspoon nutmeg

- ¼ teaspoon allspice

- three tablespoons erythritol, powdered

- 10-15 drops liquid Stevia

- 1/8 teaspoon xanthan gum

Instructions

1. Rice cauliflower in a food processor and set aside. Start heating coconut milk in a pan over medium heat.

2. Crush pecans and upload to pan over low heat to toast.

3. Add cauliflower to coconut milk, convey to a boil, and then reduce to simmer. Add spices and mix together.

4. Grind erythritol and upload to the pan, then add the stevia, flax, and chia seeds. Mix this together as exceptional you can.

5. Add cream, butter, and cream cheese to the pan and mix again. Add xanthan gum (optionally) if you need it a bit thicker.

KETO TATER TOTS

This makes a total of 36 Keto Tater Tots. Each nine piece serving comes out to be 235.75 Calories,18.65g Fats, 5.5g Net Carbs, and 9.05g Protein.

Ingredients

• 1 medium head cauliflower

• ¼ cup grated Parmesan cheese

• 2 ounces mozzarella cheese, shredded

• 1 large egg

• ½ teaspoon onion powder

• ½ teaspoon garlic powder

• 2 teaspoons psyllium husk powder

• Salt and pepper to taste

• 1 cup frying oil (I used Sir Francis Bacon Fat)

Instructions

1. Cut cauliflower head into florets. Steam till gentle. Pulse in meals processor till it resembles mashed potatoes.

2. Let cauliflower cool, then positioned into a dish cloth and wring out any extra water.

3. Add cheese, egg, and spices. Mix collectively till aggregate is thickened and may be worked with. Add 1 tsp. More psyllium husk powder at a time if wanted.

4. Roll batter into tater children, then warmth oil. Fry 6-9 at a time, flipping as they brown on each aspect.

5. Lay on paper towels to chill, then serve

ROASTED RED BELL PEPPER AND CAULIFLOWER SOUP

This makes 5 general servings of Roasted Red Bell Pepper & Cauliflower Soup. Each serving comes out to be 345 Calories, 32g Fats, 6.2g Net Carbs, and six.4g Protein.

Ingredients

• 2 Red Bell Peppers, reduce in 1/2 and de-seeded

- 1/2 head Cauliflower, cut into florets

- 2 tbsp. Duck Fat

- three medium Green Onions, diced

- three cups Chicken Broth

- 1/2 cup Heavy Cream

- four tbsp. Duck Fat

- 1 tsp. Garlic Powder

- 1 tsp. Dried Thyme

- 1 tsp. Smoked Paprika

- 1/4 tsp. Red Pepper Flakes

- four oz. Goat Cheese, crumbled (to pinnacle)

- Salt and Pepper to Taste

Instructions

1. Slice peppers in half and de-seed them. Broil for 10-15 minutes or till skin is charred and blackened. Once performed, vicinity in field with lid to steam whilst cauliflower chefs.

2. Cut cauliflower into florets and season with 2 tbsp. Melted duck fats, salt, and pepper. Roast cauliflower in 400F oven for 30-35 mins.

3. Remove the skins from the peppers by way of peeling it off carefully.

4. In a pot, bring four tbsp. Duck fat to warmness and upload diced green onion. Add seasonings into the pan to toast, then add fowl broth, purple

pepper, and cauliflower to the pan. Let this simmer for 10-20 mins.

5. Take an immersion blender to the combination. Make sure that everyone fat are emulsified. Then upload cream and mix.

6. Serve with a few crispy bacon and goats' cheese. Garnish with more thyme and inexperienced onion.

SPINACH, HERB & FETA WRAP

This makes a total of two single-serving Spinach, Herb and Feta Wraps. Each wrap comes out to be 361.5 Calories, 25.27 g Fat, 4.06 g Net Carbs, and 27.55 g Protein.

Ingredients

- five whole eggs

- three egg whites

- 1 teaspoon sesame oil

- ½ teaspoon salt

- 2 cups spinach leaves

- ½ cup crumbled feta

- 4 leaves basil, more or less chopped

- 3 complete sundried tomatoes, chopped

- Optional: 1 teaspoon olive oil

Instructions

For the Wrap

1. In a large blending bowl combine your entire eggs, egg whites, salt, and sesame oil.

2. Whisk collectively until the combination is slightly foamy. About: 30 to at least one minutes of whisking have to carry the preferred consistency.

3. Use a non-stick pan or a pan organized with cooking spray. I used a square nine ½ nonstick pan due to the fact I sense a rectangular egg wraps easier. Allow the pan to reach medium heat. Pour half of the egg combination into the skillet, cowl and decrease the heat to medium-low.

4. Once the wrap is cooked through and there's no raw egg left in the middle, take away from the pan and funky on a paper towel or plate. Prepare the second one wrap inside the same way, cooking medium-low and gradual.

For the Filling

1. Place spinach inside the skillet used for the eggs on low warmness to gently wilt the leaves. If you opt for soft leaves, go away them inside the pan for about a minute.

2. Portion out the feta, sun-dried tomatoes, basil, and oil (if using) and prepare to fill your wraps.

3. Begin with a layer of wilted spinach, observed with the feta, basil, and drizzle of oil.

4. Roll from one quit to the other. Wrap in parchment to make eating on-the-move less difficult!

VERY-VEGGIE CAULIFLOWER HASH BROWN BREAKFAST BOWL

Serves 1

Ingredients

• half of avocado

• half of lime or lemon

• garlic powder, salt, and pepper

• 2 eggs

- greater virgin olive oil

- 1-1/2 cups cauliflower rice

- 4oz mushrooms, sliced

- 1 small handful toddler spinach

- 1 inexperienced onion, chopped

- salsa

Instructions

1. Add avocado, lime or lemon juice, garlic powder, salt, and pepper to taste to a small bowl then mash with a fork and set aside. Whisk eggs with salt and pepper in a small bowl then set apart.

2. Heat a drizzle of greater virgin olive oil in a 10" skillet over medium warmth. Add mushrooms then sauté till they launch their water. After the water has cooked off, season mushrooms with garlic powder, salt, and pepper, then sauté until golden brown. Scoop into a bowl then set apart.

3. Turn warmth as much as medium-excessive then add some other drizzle of extra virgin olive oil to the skillet. Add cauliflower, season with garlic powder, salt, and pepper, then sauté until crisp-soft, 4-5 minutes. Scoop cauliflower into your serving bowl then set aside.

4. Turn warmth go into reverse to medium then add the mushrooms returned into the skillet in conjunction with the inexperienced onions and

toddler spinach. Sauté till spinach is barely wilted, 30 seconds, then add whisked eggs and scramble. Scoop mixture on top of sautéed cauliflower hash browns then top with mashed avocado and salsa.

KETO EGG FAST SNICKER DOODLE CREPES

Yield: Approximately 4 servings 1x

Ingredients

For the crepes:

- 6 eggs

- 5 ounces cream cheese, softened

- 1 tsp cinnamon

- 1 Tbsp granulated sugar replacement (Splenda, Swerve, Ideal, etc.)

- butter for frying

For the filling:

- 8 Tbsp butter, softened

- 1/3 cup granulated sugar replacement

- 1 Tbsp (or greater) cinnamon

Instructions

1. Blend all the crepe elements (except the butter) collectively in a blender or magic bullet till easy. Let the batter rest for five minutes.

2. Heat butter in a nonstick pan on medium heat till sizzling.

3. Pour enough batter into the pan to form a 6 inch crepe. Cook for about 2 mins, then turn and prepare dinner for an extra minute.

4. Remove and stack on a warm plate. You must become with approximately 8 crepes.

5. Meanwhile, blend your sweetener and cinnamon in a small bowl or baggie till combined.

6. Stir half of the mixture into your softened butter till clean.

7. To serve, spread 1 Tbsp of the butter aggregate onto the center of your crepe.

8. Roll up and sprinkle with about 1 tsp of extra sweetener/cinnamon mixture.

IBIH LOW CARB GREEN SMOOTHIE – DAIRY FREE

Yield: 6 one cup servings 1x

INGREDIENTS

- 4 cups filtered water

- 1 cup romaine lettuce

- 1/3 cup chopped fresh pineapple

- 2 Tbsp fresh parsley

- 1 Tbsp clean ginger, peeled and chopped

- 1 cup raw cucumber, peeled and sliced

- half of cup kiwi fruit, peeled and chopped

- half Hass avocado (put off pit and scoop flesh out of shell)

- 1 Tbsp granulated sugar alternative (I used Swerve)

INSTRUCTIONS

1. Combine all the components in a blender and mix until smooth. Serve bloodless. Leftovers will preserve numerous days inside the refrigerator, shake properly earlier than serving.

LOW-CARB SNAP PEA SALAD

This Low-Carb Snap Pea Salad makes a perfect

facet dish for spring.

Ingredients

- 8 oz. cauliflower riced

- 1/4 cup lemon juice

- 1/4 cup olive oil

- 1 clove garlic beaten

- 1/2 teaspoon coarse grain dijon mustard

- 1 teaspoon granulated stevia/erythritol blend

- 1/4 teaspoon pepper

- half of teaspoon sea salt

- half of cup sugar snap peas ends eliminated and each pod cut into three portions

- ¼ cup chives

- 1/2 cup sliced almonds

- ¼ cup red onions minced

Instructions

2. Pour 1 to two inches of water in a pot equipped with a steamer. Bring water to a simmer.

3. Place riced cauliflower within the steamer basket, sprinkle gently with sea salt, cover, and area over the simmering water within the

backside of the steamer. Steam till soft,

approximately 10-12 mins.

4. When cauliflower is soft, take away the

pinnacle of the steamer from the simmering

water and region it over a bowl, so any extra

water can drain out. Allow to chill, exposed for

about 10 mins, then cowl and location the

steamer and the bowl within the fridge. Chill for

as a minimum 1/2 hour or till cool to touch.

5. While cauliflower is cooling, make the

dressing. Pour olive oil in a small mixing

bowl.Gradually stream within the lemon juice

while vigorously whisking. Whisk in the garlic,

mustard, sweetener, pepper, and salt.

6. In a medium blending bowl, combine chilled cauliflower, peas, chives, almonds, and purple onions. Pour dressing over and stir to mix. Transfer to a hermetic container and refrigerate till serving. This salad is first-rate if it's far allowed to sit for some hours within the refrigerator so the flavors mingle.

CAPRESE GRILLED EGGPLANT ROLL UPS

These caprese eggplant roll usaare smooth to make and make a awesome appetizer or snack.

Prep Time- 5 mins

Cook Time- 8 minutes

Total Time- 13 mins

Servings: eight bites, approx

Ingredients

• 1 eggplant aubergine, small/medium

• 4 ozmozzarella 115g, approx

• 1 tomato large

• 2 basil leaves or a touch extra as wanted

• precise first-rate olive oil

Instructions

1. Make certain your knife is sharp before
beginning. Cut the stop off the eggplant then cut
it into skinny slices, round 0.1in/0.25cm thick
lengthwise. Discard the smaller portions which

might be specially pores and skin and now not as long from both facet.

2. Slice the mozzarella and tomato very thinly as nicely. Shred the basil leaves thinly.

3. Warm a griddle pan and lightly brush the eggplant slices with olive oil. Alternatively, drizzle on a touch and quick rub over before it's far absorbed. Place the eggplant slices on the pan and grill for a couple minutes each side. They have to soften and feature mild grill marks. As the second facet is sort of done, upload a bigger piece of mozzarella within the thick part of the eggplant slice. Top it with a slice of tomato, and upload a smaller piece of mozzarella at the thinner quit. Sprinkle over a pair pieces of basil

and drizzle a bit olive oil and a pair grinds of black

pepper, if you like. Let it prepare dinner for a

minute more than cautiously cast off from the

pan. There could be a chunk of liquid comes out

from the tomato and cheese so allow it drain off.

4. Roll the eggplant from the thinner quit, which

has handiest the cheese. You probably won't get

it to roll completely, but once it's near, keep

together with a cocktail stick. Serve warm

(better) or room temperature.

PARMESAN CAULIFLOWER STEAK

Yield: 4 Servings 1x

Ingredients

- 1 huge head cauliflower

- 4 tbsp butter

- 2 tbsp Urban Accents Manchego and Roasted

Garlic seasoning mixture

- ¼ cup parmesan cheese

- Salt and pepper to flavor

Instructions

1. Preheat oven to 400 levels

2. Remove leaves from cauliflower

3. Slice cauliflower lengthwise via center into 1

inch steaks (mine made approximately 4)

4. Melt butter in microwave and mix with seasoning blend to make paste

5. Brush mixture over steaks and season with salt and pepper to taste

6. Heat non-stick pan over medium and region cauliflower steaks for two-3 minutes till lightly browned

7. Flip cautiously, repeat

8. Place cauliflower steaks on covered baking sheet

9. Bake cauliflower steaks in oven for 15-20 minutes until golden and soft

10. Sprinkle with parmesan cheese and serve

CREAMY CILANTRO LIME COLESLAW

(LOW CARB)

Prep Time 10 minutes

Total Time 10 mins

Servings five

Ingredients

- 14 oz. coleslaw, bagged

- 1 half avocados

- ¼ cup cilantro leaves

- 2 limes, juiced

- 1 garlic clove

- ¼ cup water

• half of teaspoon salt

• cilantro to garnish

Instructions

1. In a food processor add the garlic and cilantro and method until chopped.

2. Add the lime juice, avocados and water. Pulse till excellent and creamy.

3. Take out the avocado combination and in a large bowl blend it with the coleslaw. It can be a chunk thick however it's going to cover the slaw properly.

4. For nice consequences, refrigerate for a few hours before eating to soften the cabbage.

KETO ASIAN NOODLE SALAD WITH PEANUT SAUCE

INGREDIENTS

For the salad:

- 1 cup shredded pink cabbage

- 1 cup shredded green cabbage

- 1/4 cup chopped scallions

- 1/4 cup chopped cilantro

- 4 cups shiritake noodles (tired and rinsed)

- 1/4 cup chopped peanuts

For the dressing:

- 2 tablespoons minced ginger

- 1 teaspoon minced garlic

- ½ cup filtered water

- 1 tablespoon lime juice

- 1 tablespoon toasted sesame oil

- 1 tablespoon wheat-unfastened soy sauce

- 1 tablespoon fish sauce (or coconut aminos for vegan)

- ¼ cup sugar loose peanut butter

- ¼ teaspoon cayenne pepper

- ½ teaspoon kosher salt

- 1 tablespoon granulated erythritol sweetener

INSTRUCTIONS

1. Combine all of the salad substances in a
massive bowl.

2. Combine all the dressing components in a
blender or magic bullet.

3. Blend till clean.

4. Pour the dressing over the salad and toss to
coat.

5. Serve right away, or shop in a hermetic box
inside the refrigerator for as much as 5 days. Do
not freeze.

CRUNCHY & NUTTY CAULIFLOWER SALAD

Ingredients

• three cups, 720 ml very finely chopped

cauliflower

• 1 cup, 240 ml finely chopped leek (the

inexperienced part)

• half of cup, a 120 ml chopped organic walnuts

• 1 cup, 240 ml complete-fat sour cream

• unrefined sea salt OR Himalayan salt to flavor

Instructions

1. Combine all components in a massive bowl.

Mix until properly blended.

2. Transfer into a hermetic field.

3. Refrigerate at least 3 hours earlier than serving

so that the flavors mingle and get deeper.

SPINACH ARTICHOKE SPAGHETTI SQUASH RECIPE

A healthier manner to serve a favorite dip, this

Spinach Artichoke Spaghetti Squash Recipe has

squash mixed with spinach, artichokes, and a

creamy cheese sauce.

Ingredients

• 1 spaghetti squash, seeded

• three teaspoons extra virgin olive oil

• 3/4 cup chopped onion

- 3 cloves garlic, minced

- half of cup mild bitter cream

- three oz. much less fats cream cheese

- 3/4 cup grated parmesan, divided

- 3 cups packed toddler spinach

- 1 1/4 cups canned artichoke hearts, chopped

- salt and pepper

- ¾ cup shredded mozzarella cheese

- chopped clean parsley

Instructions

1. Place the spaghetti squash in a microwave safe dish, cut side down. Pour approximately half of

an inch of water within the dish, then cover with plastic wrap and microwave till soft, about 10 minutes. Remove and permit cool slightly, then with a fork, scrape up the strings from the squash.

2. Meanwhile, in a pan, warmth the olive oil over medium warmness. Add the onion and prepare dinner until tender, five-eight minutes. Add the garlic and cook till aromatic, approximately 60 seconds. Add in the bitter cream, cream cheese and half of the parmesan cheese and stir until the cream cheese has melted and the mixture is clean. Stir inside the spinach and artichoke hearts and cook until the spinach has wilted. Season to taste with salt and pepper. Pour half of

the mixture into each spaghetti squash half and gently pull up at the spaghetti squash strings to mix with the sauce as plenty as possible. Top with the shredded mozzarella and the remaining parmesan. Place under the broiler for two-three minutes, or until the cheese is melted and bubbly.

3. Sprinkle with sparkling parsley, if desired, and serve hot.

CONCLUSION

There are many delicious plant meals which are low in carbs, but high in fats and protein.

Clearly, you do not want to be a meat eater to

acquire the benefits of low-carb eating.

CPSIA information can be obtained
at www.ICGtesting.com
Printed in the USA
BVHW041302031220
594827BV00030B/498